MW ANDERSON

Top 40 Workouts For Men Over 40

How To Lose Weight, Build Muscle & Feel Great

I have not failed. I've just found 10,000 ways that won't work.

Thomas Edison

Contents

1

Introduction

Welcome to the Top 40 Workouts For Men Over 40! I am extremely excited to be writing this book! As men over 40, we've probably come to the conclusion that unfortunately we cannot do the same things quite like we used to when we were 21. We are a little more prone to injury if we're not careful and the recovery and healing time is just a bit longer. But that's not going to stop us right?! Hell no. We get to maximize every aspect of our lives, and making health and wellness a priority helps out in so many other areas! I've certainly found that to be true with the journey I am on, which I am always looking to improve upon. We're not here for perfection, just to get a little better every day, week, month, and year!

This pocket-sized book is not one that will give you every little detail there is to know about each of the workouts. Or to go in depth about the other key components. I'm simply here to deliver the most condensed overall fitness plan, without having to flip through 100's of pages to find what you're really looking for. The popularity of each of them can vary based on your personal preferences, fitness goals, and individual health conditions. However, this is a pretty diverse list suitable for men 40 and over, regardless of where you are in your fitness journey. It consists of a mix of cardiovascular exercises, strength training, flexibility workouts, and activities that promote overall fitness and well-being. It's crucial to tailor workouts to individual fitness levels and consult with professionals when needed. (More on that later!)

This isn't necessarily a book that you have to read cover to cover (even though it's a quick read!) Rather, it's something where you can look at it first thing in the morning and jump around to a different workout each day or however often you like. It's totally up to you and what you feel like getting into that day! They are all easy to find in the table of contents. No pressure!

With that said, let's jump right in!

2

Mindset

The first few chapters are those key components I mentioned, that when paired together, can accelerate your fitness journey. I wanted to start off with a chapter on mindset because I felt it is crucial to achieving your highest possible output and a great starting point. If you're not excited about something, you're much less likely to stay engaged or even start. Ask yourself why you're doing this, even if you're just starting, haven't worked out in years, or are a regular at the gym. How good do you want to look and feel? Your mindset will certainly determine your level of success. Let's start it off positive and keep it that way. Nothing is going to happen overnight. But every day adds to that momentum, and before you know it, you're on one hell of a roll! Simply make the commitment now that I am going to make this work no matter what. You got this!

I can't move on without touching on personal development. We can be as positive as we want to be. But if what we are watching, listening to or consuming is bad or negative, it's only a matter of time before that infects our positive mindset and commitment we have made to ourselves. In addition to what we're exposing ourselves to, the people around us can certainly play a huge role in bringing us down and getting us off track. I know it's not always easy, but I highly recommend taking stock of all of those areas, and make some tough decisions on what needs to stay or go, and who needs to stay or go. You may have heard the saying that there are people you spend 5 hours with that you need to spend 5 minutes with. And there are people you spend 5 minutes with that you need to spend 5 hours with. There is a ton of great content out there, whether it be physical books, audio books, podcasts, YouTube videos, etc, that can start filling up your cup with positivity!

3

Goals

After getting the right mindset, take a little time to set some goals. What do you want to achieve in the short term? Mid-term? Long term? Get as specific as you can. Write them down every day! Whether that is first thing in the morning, before you go to bed, or both. The more you write them down and look at them, the more they'll be ingrained in your head and be at the forefront of your day-to-day life. It's also a great way to keep track of your progression and to see how far you have come. It could be a weight goal, and repetition goal, a time goal, a clothing size goal, a step goal. Whatever you want. Just get super specific! **Tip:** do this for every area of your life!

4

6 Packs Start in the Kitchen

You may or may not have heard this phrase before. But it's so true. It's pretty tough, and damn near impossible to work off a bad diet. I don't care what you're doing in the gym, a poor diet will hold you back from achieving your goals. I know when we were younger, it seemed like we could eat whatever we wanted and there wasn't nearly as much of an effect. So, what does this mean? It means you get to start making what you buy at the grocery store a priority and only buying what you need. Make a list! I find when I have a list, I get what's on it and get out of there. And when you don't bring any junk food home, it's not there to eat when you get those sudden urges! Of course, this can apply to when you're eating out, with putting in more consideration to what you're ordering and what's really all in that meal. You don't have to be a 5-star chef to come up with some basic, healthy meals. There are even some great services out there that can have clean meals delivered or all of the ingredients to make them yourselves.

Along with the food we're eating, the beverages we're consuming play a role as well. Are you making drinking water a priority? Look at what else you're drinking day to day or week to week. There are so many drinks out there that disguise themselves as good or healthy. Start looking at the ingredients! What's really in those coffee, orange juice, sodas, energy drinks, etc? Most are a sugar and artificial nightmare. Of course, we know the role that alcohol plays. The more you drink, the more likely you'll be bloated, along with the effects on your mood and energy levels. I would also recommend looking into water filtration since you will be drinking more water. That could be a standing water filter, a reverse osmosis system, and sink or shower filters. Air filters can be another great add on, especially in the winter. With not having doors and windows open very often, the air can get a little stagnant in our homes. But they are great all year round. Check the Resources section!

5

Supplements

Just a few quick things on supplements. I'm not making any recommendations or saying anything will work specifically for you. But I have found supplements to enhance my overall wellness. Getting bloodwork and your levels checked by a doctor can give you a good baseline. Some things that I have tried, or am currently using, in no particular order, that you can look into are: testosterone, whey protein, creatine, collagen, amino acids, bee pollen, magnesium, iodine, a multi vitamin, vitamin D3, zinc, B-12, and elderberry syrup. As always, getting the most pure, clean versions of these is key. When it comes to health, you can pay now, or you can certainly pay later. This is certainly something we want to be proactive in, not reactive when it may be too late. Feel free to ask some people that are farther along in their journey and are where you strive to be to see if they are using any supplements and can recommend any.

6

Accountability Partner

I have found accountability partners to be very helpful. Not just for working out, but in every area of life. We all have the best intentions when we start something new or pick something back up. But often that high level of motivation fades, leading to less interest and time devoted. Having someone to keep you motivated, accountable and on track can be a super helpful way to not lose focus and keep achieving goal after goal! Don't be afraid to ask someone. More people will be willing to support you than you think! See if one or two people will start working out with you. Maybe you can align schedules to be able to meet at least a few days a week. You're creating a win-win. You have someone to spot you, rack those weights, bounce ideas off of, keep the energy level up, get a few extra reps in, keep your goals on track and help develop more goals, and ensure you both don't quit early!

7

Stretching, Warming Up & Cooling Down

Stretching is most definitely an important part of any workout routine. While you may be able to get away without it at the very beginning doing lighter workouts, as you progress, there's no getting around it.

For me, and I'm sure a lot of men over 40, it takes a little longer to get warmed up than our younger days. I know when we were kids, we probably had no idea what stretching was or why it was needed. Depending on how intense of a workout you will be doing will determine how much of a warmup will be required. That could be a combination of stretching and then spending a few minutes on the treadmill or elliptical, or vice versa. Whatever makes you feel the most ready to do whichever workout(s) are on your list for the day!

Something that often gets overlooked is doing a proper cool down after the workout. While not as necessary early on, it could definitely help as you progress, and start doing a longer, more intense workout. Some programs or classes might have these already planned for the end. But it could be as simple as slowing down the movements, doing less and less, or finishing with some of the same stretches you started with, or a few minutes walking on the treadmill. With stretching, warming up and cooling down, you will find what works best for you as your journey moves forward!

8

Sleep & Routines

Another key component I have found to be very beneficial to me is getting the right amount of sleep. While it will vary for everyone, I prefer 7-8 hours a night. A lack of sleep can hinder our performance the next day, mentally and physically. Just think back to a time when you've been tired, and how it affected your mood and energy levels that day. I have found that keeping the room as dark as possible, blocking out any possible light from outside, clocks or electronic devices very helpful. Don't forget to put your cell phone on vibrate. And keep it at least 5 or 6 feet away from you to avoid waking up to notifications. Also figure out what temperature you sleep best at. That can have an effect on how well you sleep. I keep mine at 68 or 69 through the night.

A great compliment to getting enough sleep is keeping the same schedule/routine as many days that you can. I know for me, the more I start altering the time I get up and go to bed, the more off I feel the next day. I find the more often I can stick to getting up at the same time (within a half hour) and getting to bed at the same time (within a half hour), the more efficient I am day in and day out. Of course, there are going to be exceptions. And I'm certainly not going to say don't take part in something just for the sake of the routine! Sometimes we'll have to make adjustments for family, work, travel etc. But it's something to keep in mind for the long term.

9

The Top 40 Workouts!

Here they are, in no particular order. Pick just one to start, or feel free to combine as many as you like! Remember, a lot of the equipment listed can be rented or will already be at the gym. Don't feel like you have to run out and spend thousands of dollars. And don't forget to have fun!

1. Walking

Maybe one of the most well-known, versatile, and easiest workouts to do. You can get a walk in just about anywhere or anytime of the day, indoors or outdoors. Just a few of the possible benefits of walking are improved cardiovascular health, weight management, mental well-being, joint health, and accessibility.

What Do You Need: an athletic shoe or even just a comfortable shoe, and comfortable clothes for the conditions.

2. Jogging/Running

If you're ready to take it one step further (pun intended) from walking, you can mix in some jogging/running. Like walking, going for a jog or run can be achieved indoors and outdoors, in a variety of settings.

Some of the possible benefits of jogging and running are a higher calorie burn, cardiovascular endurance, mood enhancement, bone density, and versatility.

What Do You Need: an athletic/running shoe recommended, more athletic type clothing

3. Cycling

Cycling is a nice alternative because you can get a similar type of workout to running, but can get a lot more distance in. Again, you could do it indoors on a stationary bike, or in many outdoor settings with your bike. Some of cycling's possible benefits include lower impact on the joints, cardiovascular health, lower body strength, versatility, and weight management.

What Do You Need: an athletic shoe, athletic type clothes, a stationary bike, or an outdoor bike (road or mountain)

4. Swimming

Who doesn't love being in the water. And depending on the temperature, it can certainly wake you up! You can get a good swim at an indoor pool, or outside at a nearby open body of water. Some possible benefits are a more full-body type workout, lower impact on joints, cardiovascular endurance, flexibility, and mental well-being.

What Do You Need: a pair of swimming trunks and some goggles

5. Strength Training

This could encompass many things and many parts of the body. But with more of a focus on using weights and/or machines to start building muscle. A few possible benefits could be lean muscle mass, a metabolism boost, bone density improvement, daily functional strength, and posture and stability.

What Do You Need: athletic shoes, athletic type clothes

6. Bodyweight Exercises (e.g., Push-ups, Squats, Lunges)

A great starting point. Or it could even be a high intensity workout depending on how many sets and how fast you want to go! Ability to do this virtually anywhere, anytime, as you don't need anything. It features strength building, flexibility, convenience, improved body composition, and functional fitness.

What Do You Need: at least comfortable clothes and athletic shoes

7. Yoga

No it's not just for women! You could be a total beginner or maybe it's something you tried once and want to incorporate more. Another workout that is perfect to do anywhere, anytime at home or outside somewhere. Or lots of places offer classes. Can be great for flexibility, stress reduction, balance, muscle tone, and mind-body connection.

What Do You Need: comfortable clothes, a mat if you're doing any seated yoga

8. Pilates

While along the lines of strength training, it focuses more on improving muscle tone rather than building muscles, with similar results. Another one you can do just about anywhere while at home. And it shouldn't be hard to find classes in your area. Some benefits are core strength, posture improvement, flexibility, mindful movement, and lower impact on joints.

What Do You Need: comfortable clothes, athletic shoes, just a mat for beginners. As you advance, such things as resistance bands and light weights could be added.

9. HIIT (High-Intensity Interval Training)

While this type of workout can get pretty intense, don't be afraid to try it out at a slower pace while you get it all down. It usually consists of several rounds that alternate between several minutes of high intensity movements. You can try it at home first before jumping into a class. Can have some weights or none at all. Some benefits include efficient calorie burn, metabolic boost, cardiovascular health, time-efficiency, and fat loss.

What Do You Need: athletic shoes and clothes

10. Circuit Training

This is somewhat similar to HIIT, but circuit can vary on the amount of effort over the duration of the workout, the time to complete and periods of rest. You can do it all at home or join some local classes. Can have some weights or none at all. Benefits could be a total body workout, cardiovascular endurance, time efficiency, variety, and adaptability.

What Do You Need: athletic shoes and clothes

11. Resistance Band Workouts

Not just for stretching! Just starting out, these can help with stretching, while slowly progressing into a serious workout. Easy to do anywhere. They come in various resistance strengths. Known benefits are versatility, joint-friendly, strength building, portable, and improved flexibility.

What Do You Need: elastic resistance bands, and at least comfortable clothes and shoes

12. Kettlebell Exercises

Simply a ball with a handle at the top, they can offer a variety of exercises. And no you don't have to be an experienced weightlifter. There are online or in person classes that can take you on the whole journey. Some possible benefits are a total body workout, cardiovascular fitness, functional strength, core engagement, and increased grip strength.

What Do You Need: athletic clothes and shoes, various weighted kettlebells

13. Rowing

Not just for racing little boats! Although if you have a kayak or canoe, that's a great way to get it in. You can also usually find some rowing machines at the gym. Or you can find one you like for home use. Possible benefits could be cardiovascular endurance, lower impact on joints, muscle toning, calorie burn, and improved posture.

What Do You Need: Outside: canoe/kayak, a paddle & a body of water. Inside: athletic clothes & shoes and a rowing machine

14. Elliptical Training

A great way to warm up before another workout. Or to do a complete cardio workout, without the rigors of running. Again, these are usually a staple at the gym. Or you can get one to use at home. Some benefits could be lower impact cardio, engaging upper & lower body, versatility, calorie burn, and varying intensities.

What Do You Need: athletic clothes and shoes and an elliptical machine

15. Boxing

Don't worry. We're not fighting anyone! At first, work on your form, then move into focusing on power, speed and using a punching/heavy bag. Another workout that can be done at home or at a class. Possible benefits are cardiovascular conditioning, full-body engagement, stress relief, improved coordination, and strength building.

What Do You Need: athletic clothes and shoes, gloves if striking a punching bag

16. Tai Chi

This involves a series of slow gentle movements and physical postures, a meditative state of mind, and controlled breathing. You can learn at home or find an instructor locally to get really serious. Some benefits include stress reduction, balance improvement, joint flexibility, mind-body connection, and energy flow.

What Do You Need: loose/comfortable clothes, shoes (optional)

17. Golf (Walking the Course)

Yes you can still do that! A lot of courses should have walking carts for your clubs. Just check with the course if they do and if there are any times they don't allow walking for some reason. Due to conditions, they may ONLY allow walking. Benefits include cardiovascular exercise, low impact on joints, social interaction, improved concentration, and outdoor enjoyment.

What Do You Need: comfortable clothes, golf or athletic shoes, golf clubs, balls, tees

18. Tennis

A fun indoor or outdoor activity, that can be as light or intense as you want to make it. While courts aren't everywhere, most communities have an outdoor court, and possibly some indoor courts. You can even use a racquetball court to practice. Some benefits possible are cardiovascular fitness, improved agility, full-body workout, social engagement, and mental stimulation

What Do You Need: comfortable clothes, athletic shoes, tennis racket & balls

19. Mountain Biking

A little step up from cycling, as the terrain is unpredictable and rougher. But with some preplanning, beginners can find a modest path to tackle. Benefits could be cardiovascular endurance, lower body strength, balance and coordination, mental focus, and an enjoyable outdoor activity.

What Do You Need: comfortable clothes, athletic/hiking shoes, mountain bike

20. Trail Running/Hiking

Along the lines of mountain biking, the terrain will be more unpredictable and rougher than indoor running or running on a track. But it is certainly a great alternative and a chance to be one with nature. Possible benefits include cardiovascular exercise, joint health, mental well-being, strengthening leg muscles, and versatility.

What Do You Need: athletic/comfortable clothes, running/trail running shoes

21. Snow Skiing

Who doesn't love playing in the snow. Obviously there needs to be snow to do this. So, this might be more of a winter sport. You could try on your own. But I would recommend asking a friend who's had some experience, or getting a few lessons at a resort just to be on the safe side! A few benefits are cardiovascular exercise, lower body strength, improved balance, calorie burn, and outdoor enjoyment.

What Do You Need: skis, boots, snow attire, goggles

22. Snowboarding

Like skiing, this will be more of a winter activity. Might be a little easier to learn on your own. But if you know someone that does, definitely pick their brain to speed up the learning curve. And most ski resorts can teach you as well. Some benefits could be a full-body workout, cardiovascular fitness, enhanced flexibility, mental focus, and social interaction.

What Do You Need: a snowboard, boots, snow attire, goggles

23. Surfing

From the cold to the warm! There's nothing like riding a wave, being in the water, and at the beach. Obviously you can't do this anywhere. But if you're near a body of water that has some good waves, try it out! Benefits can be core strength, cardiovascular exercise, enhanced coordination, mindfulness, and a connection with nature.

What Do You Need: at least swim trunks, a wet suit preferred, surf board

24. Rock Climbing

An indoor or outdoor activity. For beginners, indoors would be a much easier place to start, as there will be professionals there to guide you, and you can be in a harness for safety. Get that down before trying a real mountain, unless it's not a very steep incline. Possible benefits could be full-body strength, improved flexibility, mental challenges, enhanced grip strength, and community engagement.

What Do You Need: Indoor: athletic clothes, athletic shoes; Outdoor: climbing shoes, chalk bag/chalk, harness, helmet, gloves, sunglasses

25. Functional Fitness Workouts

What the heck does that mean?! Basically, it is a type of workout geared mainly toward better function when performing our everyday tasks, like moving heavier things up high, bending to get something off of the floor, or walking up and down some stairs. Usually these can be done in a circuit format, similar to HIIT or CrossFit. A few benefits can be real-world movements, improved mobility, balanced muscle development, prevention of injuries, and adaptability.

What Do You Need: athletic clothes, athletic shoes

26. TRX Suspension Training

No, we're not working on cars here. It comes from the Navy SEALs, and stands for total resistance exercises. A great workout for beginners to advanced. You can attach the bands to a secure door, or get the wall anchor. Some benefits are a total body workout, core strength, versatility, improved flexibility, and functional fitness.

What Do You Need: athletic clothes, athletic shoes, resistance bands

27. CrossFit

On the mid to high intensity side. This would require some weights, dumbbells etc. Great for home if you have the equipment, or at a CrossFit gym. There is a learning curve at first. Benefits include high-intensity cardio, variety, community engagement, functional strength, and adaptive workouts.

What Do You Need: athletic clothes, athletic shoes, equipment if at home

28. Barre Workouts

Great for all fitness levels, it is a mix of toning, body weight exercises, and weights. Perfect to do at home or at a class led by an instructor in your local area. Possible benefits are muscle toning, improved posture, low impact on joints, flexibility, and balance enhancement.

What Do You Need: comfortable/athletic clothes, shoes optional, yoga mat

29. Stair Climbing

There are no shortages of stairs in our lives. You can do this at home, on a stair climber at the gym, or just about anywhere. Do as many or as little amount as you like, one or 2 steps at a time. Benefits are cardiovascular exercise, lower body strength, calorie burn, accessible exercise, and versatility.

What Do You Need: comfortable/athletic clothes, athletic shoes

30. Zumba

Whether you like to dance or not, Zumba will get you in the zone. It usually mixes some Latin and international music with some aerobic training. Perfect for any level, at home or at a local class. Some benefits are calorie burning, cardiovascular fitness, stress relief, improved coordination, and social interaction.

What Do You Need: comfortable clothes, athletic shoes

31. Kickboxing

Again, don't worry, we're not fighting anyone! Taking it farther than just boxing, this is great for anyone. It adds in kicking air and bags. Beginners can benefit from being at a local class led by an instructor. Included benefits are cardiovascular conditioning, full-body workout, calorie burn, stress relief, and improved coordination.

What Do You Need: comfortable/athletic clothes, gloves if using a bag

32. Bodybuilding

If you are looking to take it past just toning and working the whole body, and really pack on some muscle, it is definitely possible at our age. While you can do it by yourself, it's helpful to have a partner to spot and push you. Just be prepared to buy some new clothes! Possible benefits could be muscle development, metabolism boost, bone health, improved body composition, and mental discipline.

What Do You Need: athletic clothes, athletic shoes; gloves, chalk, straps weight belt possibly

33. Aerobics

This can be one or 2 things or a larger combination of workouts. Basically, anything that gets you moving for a prolonged period of time! Take some things from this list. Or most gyms/fitness centers offer aerobics classes. Those benefits are cardiovascular fitness, weight management, mood enhancement, increased stamina, and adaptability.

What Do You Need: depends on which activity/activities you're doing

34. Water Aerobics

Taking everything aerobics into the pool! With usually an emphasis on cardio and strength training. Great to do somewhere with a pool and/or at a class, which should have all of the needed equipment. Possible benefits are low-impact exercise, resistance training, cardiovascular conditioning, cooling effect, social interaction.

What Do You Need: swim trunks

35. Body Combat

Nope still no fighting! This is a martial art inspired workout, kicking and punching, but with a mix of boxing, karate, taekwondo, kung fu, capoeira, and muay thai. Benefits possible are cardiovascular fitness, full-body conditioning, calorie burn, stress relief, and improved coordination.

What Do You Need: comfortable clothes, athletic shoes

36. Rebounding (Mini Trampoline)

Great for any level, at home, or if there is a local class. The moves can be fast or slow, and vigorous or low intensity. Some benefits are low-impact exercise, cardiovascular fitness, improved lymphatic system function, muscle toning & strength, and enhanced balance.

What Do You Need: comfortable clothes, mini trampoline

37. Jump Rope

Not just for kids at recess! Perfect for any level, and can do it just about anywhere. See how many you can do in a row. Possible benefits could be cardiovascular fitness, calorie burn, improved coordination, full-body workout, and convenience.

What Do You Need: comfortable clothes, athletic shoes, jump rope

38. Martial Arts (e.g., Karate, Jiu-Jitsu, Taekwondo, Muay Thai)

While body combat encompasses all of these at once, it can be beneficial to take each of these on their own. Would recommend signing up for a few classes with an instructor to see if you like it. Known benefits are cardiovascular exercise, self-defense skills, improved discipline, enhanced coordination, and stress reduction.

What Do You Need: comfortable clothes

39. Paddle Boarding

Not quite like surfing, as we can do it on much calmer waters, and we are standing up. More places are renting the equipment. Great for all levels. Benefits can be core strengthening, low-impact exercise, cardiovascular health, enhanced balance, and mindful relaxation.

What Do You Need: swim trunks, paddle board & paddle

40. Mobility Exercises

This is more than just stretching. It can be a combo of yoga, stretching, agility exercises, myofascial releases, and whatever helps you move better. You can find some programs online or offered locally. Benefits could be improved flexibility, enhanced joint health, injury prevention, better posture, and increased range of motion.

What Do You Need: comfortable clothes, athletic shoes

Hiring Coaches

No matter where you are in your fitness journey, seeking the guidance of an expert coach can accelerate you getting to your goals. Not only can they help hold you accountable, but they can answer questions and tailor the best plan for you. This doesn't just apply to the fitness side of things, or incorporating the best diet. But really anywhere in life where you want to take things to the next level – business, career, relationships, etc. Look for someone that has achieved the kinds of success you want, ask lots of questions, and make sure it's a win-win for everyone! Don't be afraid to interview several before making your choice. Getting recommendations from friends and people you trust is a great way to start. In anything I have done, having a coach and/or mentor guiding me along has always resulted in a better experience and faster growth than not having one.

11

Conclusion: You Got This!

There it is! The Top 40 Workouts For Men Over 40. Hopefully it has sparked many ideas related to workouts and everything that is related to health and wellness. They truly do work so well together. Wherever you are in your health and wellness journey, I wish you nothing but the best. You can totally do this. Age is just a number. I believe 100% in you! You just have to stay committed. I really hope you've enjoyed this book as much as I've enjoyed writing it!

If you found this book helpful, I would be very appreciative if you left a favorable review for it on Amazon!

12

Resources

CPT, A. M. W., & CPT, C. S. (2023, November 10). The 24 best stretching exercises for better Flexibility. SELF. https://www.self.com/gallery/essential-stretches-slideshow

Suni, E., & Suni, E. (2023, December 8). Mastering Sleep Hygiene: Your path to quality sleep. Sleep Foundation. https://www.sleepfoundation.org/sleep-hygiene

Ascm-Cep, L. W. M. (2021, November 29). Should you try dance fitness? Verywell Fit. https://www.verywellfit.com/dance-fitness-4014009#:~:text=Cardio%2DBased%20Dance%20Fitness&text=Styles%20like%20Zumba%2C%20Jazzercise%2C%20LaBlast,all%20fall%20into%20this%20category.

Hopkins, T. (2024, January 3). 14 Best meal delivery services 2024, according to Bon Appétit Editors. Bon Appétit. https://www.bonappetit.com/story/best-meal-delivery-services

Lascano, K. (2023, June 6). 16 different types of martial arts. Gymdesk.

https://gymdesk.com/blog/different-types-of-martial-arts/

What is CrossFit? And can you do it? Here's what you need to know. (2019b, November 8). NBC News. https://www.nbcnews.com/better/lifestyle/what-crossfit-it-right-you-here-s-what-you-need-ncna1070886

Z, T. (2023, July 30). 20 TRX exercises to do with a suspension trainer + workouts. TRX Training - United States. https://www.trxtraining.com/blogs/news/trx-exercises

Amazon Self-Help Best Sellers: https://www.amazon.com/Best-Sellers-Books-Self-Help/zgbs/books/4736/ref=zg_bs_nav_books_1
   Water filters: https://prooneusa.com/
   Air filters: https://alexapure.com/collections/air-filtration